THE BEST LIFE DIET
Daily Journal

BOB GREENE

THE BEST LIFE DIET

Daily Journal

SIMON & SCHUSTER

NEW YORK   LONDON   TORONTO   SYDNEY

SIMON & SCHUSTER
Rockefeller Center
1230 Avenue of the Americas
New York, NY 10020

For information regarding special discounts for bulk purchases,
please contact Simon & Schuster Special Sales at 1-800-456-6798
or business@simonandschuster.com.

Designed by Joel Avirom and Jason Snyder

Manufactured in the United States of America

10 9 8 7 6 5 4 3 2 1

ISBN-13: 978-1-4165-4314-5
ISBN-13:   1-4165-4314-7

THE BEST LIFE DIET

Daily Journal

Introduction

Transforming your body is best accomplished when you lead an active life, follow a sound eating plan, and have the motivation and discipline to follow that plan of action. *The Best Life Diet Daily Journal* is designed to work as a companion to *The Best Life Diet*. This valuable tool can help you track your eating and exercise goals and help you better understand and control your hunger throughout the different phases of your program. The principles of the Best Life diet have shown dramatic results for countless individuals and will offer you those same results when followed consistently. *The Best Life Diet* is currently available in bookstores or online at www.thebestlife.com. Before you begin the Best Life diet plan, be sure to record your starting weight, blood pressure, total cholesterol, HDL cholesterol, LDL cholesterol, blood sugar (glucose level), and any body circumference measurement that you wish to record. Having a permanent record of these starting numbers is important, not only to ensure a safe and effective program but because seeing these numbers improve can be very motivating—and they will improve!

To log your daily entries, simply record the date and what week and day of the program you're currently at, your activity level (0–5), and all of the information that applies to your eating and exercise goals in the appropriate spaces. I also think it's important to record any eating "episodes." These can be instances that are positive in nature, such as when you encounter a situation where you would typically overindulge and don't, or negative experiences, such as eating due to emotional turmoil. There is plenty of space dedicated for this journaling for each individual day. Don't forget to record the time of each episode and any pertinent information related to it. Recording this information can be enormously helpful for discovering patterns related to emotional eating and your behavior in general. Ultimately, this journal will help you to channel your energy toward healthy journaling, thus bringing you fulfillment as you explore ways to improve your life instead of overeating.

For additional support, be sure to read *The Best Life Diet* and log onto the supporting website at www.thebestlife.com.

General Health Information

(Consult with your physician before beginning this program.)

BEFORE

Weight _____ BLOOD PRESSURE: Systolic _____ Diastolic _____

Total Cholesterol _____ LDL _____ HDL _____ Blood Glucose _____

MEASUREMENTS (OPTIONAL): Chest _____ Waist _____ Hips _____

NOTES _____

_____

_____

_____

_____

_____

_____

_____

_____

_____

_____

_____

_____

AFTER

Weight _____ BLOOD PRESSURE: Systolic _____ Diastolic _____

Total Cholesterol _____ LDL _____ HDL _____ Blood Glucose _____

MEASUREMENTS (OPTIONAL): Chest _____ Waist _____ Hips _____

NOTES _____

_____

_____

_____

_____

_____

_____

_____

_____

_____

_____

_____

_____

Goals

GOALS FOR PHASE ONE

- ► Increase your activity level.

- ► Stop eating at least two hours before bedtime.

- ► Eat three meals and at least one snack daily.

- ► Stay fully hydrated.

- ► Eliminate alcohol (for now).

- ► Bolster your diet with daily supplements.

GOALS FOR PHASE TWO

Continue the changes you made in Phase One:

- ▷ *Increase your activity level.*

- ▷ *Stop eating at least two hours before bedtime.*

- ▷ *Eat three meals and at least one snack daily.*

- ▷ *Stay fully hydrated.*

- ▷ *Eliminate alcohol (for now).*

- ▷ *Bolster your diet with daily supplements.*

- ► Increase your activity at least one level.

- ► Understand the physical nature of your hunger.

- ► Understand the emotional nature of your hunger.

- ► Use the hunger scale.

- ► Eat reasonable portions.

- ► Remove six unhealthy foods from your diet.

Build on the changes you made in Phases One and Two. If you need to, continue weight loss:

> ▷ *Live an active life.*
>
> ▷ *Eat three meals and at least one snack daily.*
>
> ▷ *Stop eating at least two hours before bedtime.*
>
> ▷ *Stay hydrated.*
>
> ▷ *Bolster your diet with daily supplements.*
>
> ▷ *Understand the physical nature of your hunger.*
>
> ▷ *Understand the emotional nature of your hunger.*
>
> ▷ *Use the hunger scale.*
>
> ▷ *Eat reasonable portions.*
>
> ▷ *Remove six unhealthy foods from your diet.*

- ▶ Increase your activity at least one level (optional).
- ▶ Introduce Anything Goes calories into your regimen.
- ▶ Balance your diet; don't exceed your maximums.
- ▶ Remove more unhealthy foods from your diet.
- ▶ Add more wholesome foods to your diet.

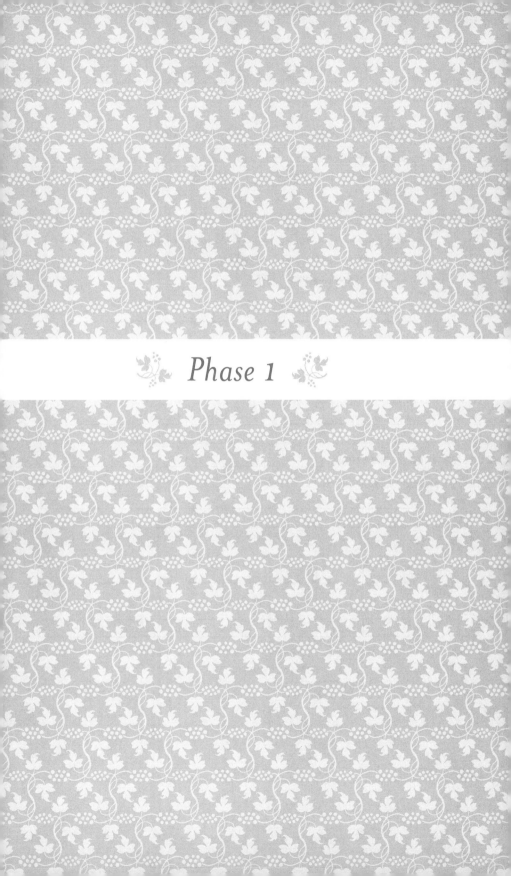

Phase 1

ACTIVITY LEVEL: 0   1   2   3   4   5

Did you eat three meals and at least one snack, including a nutritious breakfast?   Y   N

NOTES_____

_____

Eating cutoff time: ____:____   Bedtime: ____:____

Did you cut off eating at least two hours before bedtime?   Y   N

NOTES_____

_____

Did you drink at least six 8-ounce glasses of water?   Y   N

NOTES_____

_____

Did you abstain from alcohol?   Y   N

NOTES_____

_____

Did you take your vitamin supplements?   Y   N

NOTES_____

_____

Aerobic minutes or steps/day _____

Did you meet your goal?   Y   N

NOTES_____

_____

STRENGTH TRAINING

Exercise								
Weight								
Reps								
Sets								

ACTIVITY LEVEL:　　0　1　2　3　4　5

Did you eat three meals and at least one snack, including a nutritious breakfast?　　　Y　N
NOTES_____

_____

Eating cutoff time: ____:____　　　　Bedtime: ____:____
Did you cut off eating at least two hours before bedtime?　　　Y　N
NOTES_____

_____

Did you drink at least six 8-ounce glasses of water?　　　Y　N
NOTES_____

_____

Did you abstain from alcohol?　　　Y　N
NOTES_____

_____

Did you take your vitamin supplements?　　　Y　N
NOTES_____

_____

Aerobic minutes or steps/day _____
Did you meet your goal?　　　Y　N
NOTES_____

_____

STRENGTH TRAINING

Exercise								
Weight								
Reps								
Sets								

ACTIVITY LEVEL: 0   1   2   3   4   5

Did you eat three meals and at least one snack, including a nutritious breakfast?   Y   N
NOTES _____
_____

Eating cutoff time: ____:____   Bedtime: ____:____
Did you cut off eating at least two hours before bedtime?   Y   N
NOTES _____
_____

Did you drink at least six 8-ounce glasses of water?   Y   N
NOTES _____
_____

Did you abstain from alcohol?   Y   N
NOTES _____
_____

Did you take your vitamin supplements?   Y   N
NOTES _____
_____

Aerobic minutes or steps/day _____
Did you meet your goal?   Y   N
NOTES _____
_____

STRENGTH TRAINING

Exercise								
Weight								
Reps								
Sets								

ACTIVITY LEVEL: 0   1   2   3   4   5

Did you eat three meals and at least one snack, including a nutritious breakfast?   Y   N
NOTES_____
_____

Eating cutoff time: ____:____   Bedtime: ____:____
Did you cut off eating at least two hours before bedtime?   Y   N
NOTES_____
_____

Did you drink at least six 8-ounce glasses of water?   Y   N
NOTES_____
_____

Did you abstain from alcohol?   Y   N
NOTES_____
_____

Did you take your vitamin supplements?   Y   N
NOTES_____
_____

Aerobic minutes or steps/day _____
Did you meet your goal?   Y   N
NOTES_____
_____

STRENGTH TRAINING

Exercise								
Weight								
Reps								
Sets								

WEEK: **DATE:** **PHASE 1**

ACTIVITY LEVEL: 0   1   2   3   4   5

Did you eat three meals and at least one snack, including a nutritious breakfast?   Y   N
NOTES_____
_____

Eating cutoff time: ____:____   Bedtime: ____:____
Did you cut off eating at least two hours before bedtime?   Y   N
NOTES_____
_____

Did you drink at least six 8-ounce glasses of water?   Y   N
NOTES_____
_____

Did you abstain from alcohol?   Y   N
NOTES_____
_____

Did you take your vitamin supplements?   Y   N
NOTES_____
_____

Aerobic minutes or steps/day _____
Did you meet your goal?   Y   N
NOTES_____
_____

STRENGTH TRAINING

Exercise								
Weight								
Reps								
Sets								

ACTIVITY LEVEL: 0   1   2   3   4   5

Did you eat three meals and at least one snack, including a nutritious breakfast?   Y   N
NOTES_____
_____

Eating cutoff time: ____:____   Bedtime: ____:____
Did you cut off eating at least two hours before bedtime?   Y   N
NOTES_____
_____

Did you drink at least six 8-ounce glasses of water?   Y   N
NOTES_____
_____

Did you abstain from alcohol?   Y   N
NOTES_____
_____

Did you take your vitamin supplements?   Y   N
NOTES_____
_____

Aerobic minutes or steps/day _____
Did you meet your goal?   Y   N
NOTES_____
_____

STRENGTH TRAINING

Exercise								
Weight								
Reps								
Sets								

ACTIVITY LEVEL: 0   1   2   3   4   5

Did you eat three meals and at least one snack, including a nutritious breakfast?   Y   N
NOTES _____
_____

Eating cutoff time: ____:____   Bedtime: ____:____
Did you cut off eating at least two hours before bedtime?   Y   N
NOTES _____
_____

Did you drink at least six 8-ounce glasses of water?   Y   N
NOTES _____
_____

Did you abstain from alcohol?   Y   N
NOTES _____
_____

Did you take your vitamin supplements?   Y   N
NOTES _____
_____

Aerobic minutes or steps/day _____
Did you meet your goal?   Y   N
NOTES _____
_____

STRENGTH TRAINING

Exercise								
Weight								
Reps								
Sets								

Weekly Summary

How many days did you eat three meals and at least one snack?   _____

How many days did you cut off your eating at least two hours before bedtime?   _____

How many days did you drink at least six 8-ounce glasses of water?   _____

How many days did you abstain from alcohol?   _____

How many days did you take your vitamin supplements?   _____

Total aerobic minutes/steps for the week   _____

Did you meet your aerobic/step goal?   Y   N

Did you meet your strength training goals for the week?   Y   N

How was your week overall? _____

_____

ACTIVITY LEVEL: 0 1 2 3 4 5

Did you eat three meals and at least one snack, including a nutritious breakfast? Y N

NOTES_____

_____

Eating cutoff time: ____:____ Bedtime: ____:____

Did you cut off eating at least two hours before bedtime? Y N

NOTES_____

_____

Did you drink at least six 8-ounce glasses of water? Y N

NOTES_____

_____

Did you abstain from alcohol? Y N

NOTES_____

_____

Did you take your vitamin supplements? Y N

NOTES_____

_____

Aerobic minutes or steps/day _____

Did you meet your goal? Y N

NOTES_____

_____

STRENGTH TRAINING

Exercise								
Weight								
Reps								
Sets								

ACTIVITY LEVEL: 0   1   2   3   4   5

Did you eat three meals and at least one snack, including a nutritious breakfast?   Y   N
NOTES _____

_____

Eating cutoff time: ____:____   Bedtime: ____:____
Did you cut off eating at least two hours before bedtime?   Y   N
NOTES _____

_____

Did you drink at least six 8-ounce glasses of water?   Y   N
NOTES _____

_____

Did you abstain from alcohol?   Y   N
NOTES _____

_____

Did you take your vitamin supplements?   Y   N
NOTES _____

_____

Aerobic minutes or steps/day _____
Did you meet your goal?   Y   N
NOTES _____

_____

STRENGTH TRAINING

Exercise								
Weight								
Reps								
Sets								

ACTIVITY LEVEL: 0   1   2   3   4   5

Did you eat three meals and at least one snack, including a nutritious breakfast?   Y   N
NOTES _____
_____

Eating cutoff time: ___ : ___   Bedtime: ___ : ___
Did you cut off eating at least two hours before bedtime?   Y   N
NOTES _____
_____

Did you drink at least six 8-ounce glasses of water?   Y   N
NOTES _____
_____

Did you abstain from alcohol?   Y   N
NOTES _____
_____

Did you take your vitamin supplements?   Y   N
NOTES _____
_____

Aerobic minutes or steps/day _____
Did you meet your goal?   Y   N
NOTES _____
_____

STRENGTH TRAINING

Exercise								
Weight								
Reps								
Sets								

WEEK: **DATE:**   **PHASE 1**

ACTIVITY LEVEL: 0   1   2   3   4   5

Did you eat three meals and at least one snack, including a nutritious breakfast?   Y   N
NOTES _____
_____

Eating cutoff time: ____:____   Bedtime: ____:____

Did you cut off eating at least two hours before bedtime?   Y   N
NOTES _____
_____

Did you drink at least six 8-ounce glasses of water?   Y   N
NOTES _____
_____

Did you abstain from alcohol?   Y   N
NOTES _____
_____

Did you take your vitamin supplements?   Y   N
NOTES _____
_____

Aerobic minutes or steps/day _____

Did you meet your goal?   Y   N
NOTES _____
_____

STRENGTH TRAINING

Exercise								
Weight								
Reps								
Sets								

ACTIVITY LEVEL: 0 1 2 3 4 5

Did you eat three meals and at least one snack, including a nutritious breakfast?   Y   N

NOTES _____

_____

Eating cutoff time: ____:____   Bedtime: ____:____

Did you cut off eating at least two hours before bedtime?   Y   N

NOTES _____

_____

Did you drink at least six 8-ounce glasses of water?   Y   N

NOTES _____

_____

Did you abstain from alcohol?   Y   N

NOTES _____

_____

Did you take your vitamin supplements?   Y   N

NOTES _____

_____

Aerobic minutes or steps/day _____

Did you meet your goal?   Y   N

NOTES _____

_____

STRENGTH TRAINING

Exercise								
Weight								
Reps								
Sets								

ACTIVITY LEVEL: 0   1   2   3   4   5

Did you eat three meals and at least one snack, including a nutritious breakfast?   Y   N
NOTES _____
_____

Eating cutoff time: ____:____   Bedtime: ____:____
Did you cut off eating at least two hours before bedtime?   Y   N
NOTES _____
_____

Did you drink at least six 8-ounce glasses of water?   Y   N
NOTES _____
_____

Did you abstain from alcohol?   Y   N
NOTES _____
_____

Did you take your vitamin supplements?   Y   N
NOTES _____
_____

Aerobic minutes or steps/day _____
Did you meet your goal?   Y   N
NOTES _____
_____

STRENGTH TRAINING

Exercise								
Weight								
Reps								
Sets								

ACTIVITY LEVEL: 0   1   2   3   4   5

Did you eat three meals and at least one snack, including a nutritious breakfast?   Y   N
NOTES _____
_____

Eating cutoff time: ____:____   Bedtime: ____:____
Did you cut off eating at least two hours before bedtime?   Y   N
NOTES _____
_____

Did you drink at least six 8-ounce glasses of water?   Y   N
NOTES _____
_____

Did you abstain from alcohol?   Y   N
NOTES _____
_____

Did you take your vitamin supplements?   Y   N
NOTES _____
_____

Aerobic minutes or steps/day _____
Did you meet your goal?   Y   N
NOTES _____
_____

STRENGTH TRAINING

Exercise								
Weight								
Reps								
Sets								

Weekly Summary

How many days did you eat three meals and at least one snack?   _____

How many days did you cut off your eating at least two hours before bedtime?   _____

How many days did you drink at least six 8-ounce glasses of water?   _____

How many days did you abstain from alcohol?   _____

How many days did you take your vitamin supplements?   _____

Total aerobic minutes/steps for the week   _____

Did you meet your aerobic/step goal?   Y   N

Did you meet your strength training goals for the week?   Y   N

How was your week overall? _____

_____

_____

_____

_____

_____

_____

_____

_____

_____

_____

_____

_____

_____

_____

_____

_____

_____

_____

_____

_____

_____

_____

ACTIVITY LEVEL: 0   1   2   3   4   5

Did you eat three meals and at least one snack, including a nutritious breakfast?   Y   N
NOTES_____
_____

Eating cutoff time: ___:___   Bedtime: ___:___
Did you cut off eating at least two hours before bedtime?   Y   N
NOTES_____
_____

Did you drink at least six 8-ounce glasses of water?   Y   N
NOTES_____
_____

Did you abstain from alcohol?   Y   N
NOTES_____
_____

Did you take your vitamin supplements?   Y   N
NOTES_____
_____

Aerobic minutes or steps/day _____
Did you meet your goal?   Y   N
NOTES_____
_____

STRENGTH TRAINING

Exercise								
Weight								
Reps								
Sets								

ACTIVITY LEVEL: 0   1   2   3   4   5

Did you eat three meals and at least one snack, including a nutritious breakfast?   Y   N
NOTES_____
_____

Eating cutoff time: ___:___   Bedtime: ___:___
Did you cut off eating at least two hours before bedtime?   Y   N
NOTES_____
_____

Did you drink at least six 8-ounce glasses of water?   Y   N
NOTES_____
_____

Did you abstain from alcohol?   Y   N
NOTES_____
_____

Did you take your vitamin supplements?   Y   N
NOTES_____
_____

Aerobic minutes or steps/day _____
Did you meet your goal?   Y   N
NOTES_____
_____

STRENGTH TRAINING

Exercise							
Weight							
Reps							
Sets							

ACTIVITY LEVEL: 0   1   2   3   4   5

Did you eat three meals and at least one snack, including a nutritious breakfast?   Y   N

NOTES _____

_____

Eating cutoff time: ____:____   Bedtime: ____:____

Did you cut off eating at least two hours before bedtime?   Y   N

NOTES _____

_____

Did you drink at least six 8-ounce glasses of water?   Y   N

NOTES _____

_____

Did you abstain from alcohol?   Y   N

NOTES _____

_____

Did you take your vitamin supplements?   Y   N

NOTES _____

_____

Aerobic minutes or steps/day _____

Did you meet your goal?   Y   N

NOTES _____

_____

STRENGTH TRAINING

Exercise								
Weight								
Reps								
Sets								

ACTIVITY LEVEL: 0 1 2 3 4 5

Did you eat three meals and at least one snack, including a nutritious breakfast? Y N

NOTES _____

_____

Eating cutoff time: ___:___   Bedtime: ___:___

Did you cut off eating at least two hours before bedtime? Y N

NOTES _____

_____

Did you drink at least six 8-ounce glasses of water? Y N

NOTES _____

_____

Did you abstain from alcohol? Y N

NOTES _____

_____

Did you take your vitamin supplements? Y N

NOTES _____

_____

Aerobic minutes or steps/day _____

Did you meet your goal? Y N

NOTES _____

_____

STRENGTH TRAINING

Exercise								
Weight								
Reps								
Sets								

ACTIVITY LEVEL: 0 1 2 3 4 5

Did you eat three meals and at least one snack, including a nutritious breakfast?   Y N
NOTES_____
_____

Eating cutoff time: ___:___   Bedtime: ___:___
Did you cut off eating at least two hours before bedtime?   Y N
NOTES_____
_____

Did you drink at least six 8-ounce glasses of water?   Y N
NOTES_____
_____

Did you abstain from alcohol?   Y N
NOTES_____
_____

Did you take your vitamin supplements?   Y N
NOTES_____
_____

Aerobic minutes or steps/day _____
Did you meet your goal?   Y N
NOTES_____
_____

STRENGTH TRAINING

Exercise								
Weight								
Reps								
Sets								

ACTIVITY LEVEL: 0   1   2   3   4   5

Did you eat three meals and at least one snack, including a nutritious breakfast?   Y   N
NOTES _____

_____

Eating cutoff time: ___:___   Bedtime: ___:___
Did you cut off eating at least two hours before bedtime?   Y   N
NOTES _____

_____

Did you drink at least six 8-ounce glasses of water?   Y   N
NOTES _____

_____

Did you abstain from alcohol?   Y   N
NOTES _____

_____

Did you take your vitamin supplements?   Y   N
NOTES _____

_____

Aerobic minutes or steps/day _____
Did you meet your goal?   Y   N
NOTES _____

_____

STRENGTH TRAINING

Exercise								
Weight								
Reps								
Sets								

ACTIVITY LEVEL: 0   1   2   3   4   5

Did you eat three meals and at least one snack, including a nutritious breakfast?   Y   N
NOTES _____
_____

Eating cutoff time: ___:___   Bedtime: ___:___
Did you cut off eating at least two hours before bedtime?   Y   N
NOTES _____
_____

Did you drink at least six 8-ounce glasses of water?   Y   N
NOTES _____
_____

Did you abstain from alcohol?   Y   N
NOTES _____
_____

Did you take your vitamin supplements?   Y   N
NOTES _____
_____

Aerobic minutes or steps/day _____
Did you meet your goal?   Y   N
NOTES _____
_____

STRENGTH TRAINING

Exercise								
Weight								
Reps								
Sets								

Weekly Summary

How many days did you eat three meals and at least one snack? _____

How many days did you cut off your eating at least two hours before bedtime? _____

How many days did you drink at least six 8-ounce glasses of water? _____

How many days did you abstain from alcohol? _____

How many days did you take your vitamin supplements? _____

Total aerobic minutes/steps for the week _____

Did you meet your aerobic/step goal?   Y   N

Did you meet your strength training goals for the week?   Y   N

How was your week overall? _____

_____

_____

_____

ACTIVITY LEVEL: 0   1   2   3   4   5

Did you eat three meals and at least one snack, including a nutritious breakfast?   Y   N

NOTES _____

_____

Eating cutoff time: ____:____   Bedtime: ____:____

Did you cut off eating at least two hours before bedtime?   Y   N

NOTES _____

_____

Did you drink at least six 8-ounce glasses of water?   Y   N

NOTES _____

_____

Did you abstain from alcohol?   Y   N

NOTES _____

_____

Did you take your vitamin supplements?   Y   N

NOTES _____

_____

Aerobic minutes or steps/day _____

Did you meet your goal?   Y   N

NOTES _____

_____

STRENGTH TRAINING

Exercise								
Weight								
Reps								
Sets								

ACTIVITY LEVEL: 0   1   2   3   4   5

Did you eat three meals and at least one snack, including a nutritious breakfast?   Y   N
NOTES_____

_____

Eating cutoff time: ____:____   Bedtime: ____:____

Did you cut off eating at least two hours before bedtime?   Y   N
NOTES_____

_____

Did you drink at least six 8-ounce glasses of water?   Y   N
NOTES_____

_____

Did you abstain from alcohol?   Y   N
NOTES_____

_____

Did you take your vitamin supplements?   Y   N
NOTES_____

_____

Aerobic minutes or steps/day _____

Did you meet your goal?   Y   N
NOTES_____

_____

STRENGTH TRAINING

Exercise								
Weight								
Reps								
Sets								

ACTIVITY LEVEL:　　0　1　2　3　4　5

Did you eat three meals and at least one snack, including a nutritious breakfast?　　Y　N
NOTES _____

_____

Eating cutoff time: ____:____　　　　Bedtime: ____:____

Did you cut off eating at least two hours before bedtime?　　Y　N
NOTES _____

_____

Did you drink at least six 8-ounce glasses of water?　　Y　N
NOTES _____

_____

Did you abstain from alcohol?　　Y　N
NOTES _____

_____

Did you take your vitamin supplements?　　Y　N
NOTES _____

_____

Aerobic minutes or steps/day _____

Did you meet your goal?　　Y　N
NOTES _____

_____

STRENGTH TRAINING

Exercise								
Weight								
Reps								
Sets								

ACTIVITY LEVEL: 0 1 2 3 4 5

Did you eat three meals and at least one snack, including a nutritious breakfast?   Y N

NOTES _____

_____

Eating cutoff time: ____:____   Bedtime: ____:____

Did you cut off eating at least two hours before bedtime?   Y N

NOTES _____

_____

Did you drink at least six 8-ounce glasses of water?   Y N

NOTES _____

_____

Did you abstain from alcohol?   Y N

NOTES _____

_____

Did you take your vitamin supplements?   Y N

NOTES _____

_____

Aerobic minutes or steps/day _____

Did you meet your goal?   Y N

NOTES _____

_____

STRENGTH TRAINING

Exercise								
Weight								
Reps								
Sets								

ACTIVITY LEVEL: 0   1   2   3   4   5

Did you eat three meals and at least one snack, including a nutritious breakfast?   Y   N
NOTES_____

_____

Eating cutoff time: ____:____   Bedtime: ____:____
Did you cut off eating at least two hours before bedtime?   Y   N
NOTES_____

_____

Did you drink at least six 8-ounce glasses of water?   Y   N
NOTES_____

_____

Did you abstain from alcohol?   Y   N
NOTES_____

_____

Did you take your vitamin supplements?   Y   N
NOTES_____

_____

Aerobic minutes or steps/day _____
Did you meet your goal?   Y   N
NOTES_____

_____

STRENGTH TRAINING

Exercise								
Weight								
Reps								
Sets								

ACTIVITY LEVEL: 0   1   2   3   4   5

Did you eat three meals and at least one snack, including a nutritious breakfast?   Y   N

NOTES _____

_____

Eating cutoff time: ____:____   Bedtime: ____:____

Did you cut off eating at least two hours before bedtime?   Y   N

NOTES _____

_____

Did you drink at least six 8-ounce glasses of water?   Y   N

NOTES _____

_____

Did you abstain from alcohol?   Y   N

NOTES _____

_____

Did you take your vitamin supplements?   Y   N

NOTES _____

_____

Aerobic minutes or steps/day _____

Did you meet your goal?   Y   N

NOTES _____

_____

STRENGTH TRAINING

Exercise								
Weight								
Reps								
Sets								

ACTIVITY LEVEL: 0   1   2   3   4   5

Did you eat three meals and at least one snack, including a nutritious breakfast?   Y   N
NOTES_____
_____

Eating cutoff time: ___:___   Bedtime: ___:___
Did you cut off eating at least two hours before bedtime?   Y   N
NOTES_____
_____

Did you drink at least six 8-ounce glasses of water?   Y   N
NOTES_____
_____

Did you abstain from alcohol?   Y   N
NOTES_____
_____

Did you take your vitamin supplements?   Y   N
NOTES_____
_____

Aerobic minutes or steps/day _____
Did you meet your goal?   Y   N
NOTES_____
_____

STRENGTH TRAINING

Exercise								
Weight								
Reps								
Sets								

Weekly Summary

How many days did you eat three meals and at least one snack? _____

How many days did you cut off your eating at least two hours before bedtime? _____

How many days did you drink at least six 8-ounce glasses of water? _____

How many days did you abstain from alcohol? _____

How many days did you take your vitamin supplements? _____

Total aerobic minutes/steps for the week _____

Did you meet your aerobic/step goal?   Y   N

Did you meet your strength training goals for the week?   Y   N

How was your week overall? _____

_____

_____

_____

_____

_____

_____

_____

_____

_____

_____

_____

_____

_____

_____

_____

_____

_____

_____

_____

_____

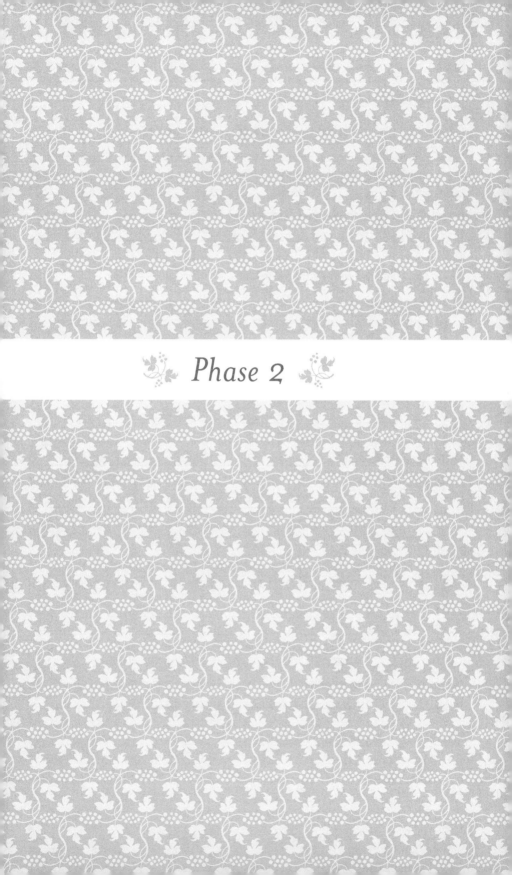

Phase 2

ACTIVITY LEVEL: 0   1   2   3   4   5

Did you eat three meals and at least one snack, including a nutritious breakfast?   Y   N
NOTES _____
_____

Eating cutoff time: ____:____   Bedtime: ____:____
Did you cut off eating at least two hours before bedtime?   Y   N
NOTES _____
_____

Did you drink at least six 8-ounce glasses of water?   Y   N
NOTES _____
_____

Did you abstain from alcohol?   Y   N
NOTES _____
_____

Did you take your vitamin supplements?   Y   N
NOTES _____
_____

Aerobic minutes or steps/day _____
Did you meet your goal?   Y   N
NOTES _____
_____

STRENGTH TRAINING

Exercise								
Weight								
Reps								
Sets								

Breakfast   ____:____   Hunger rating before eating ____ Hunger rating after eating ____

Lunch   ____:____   Hunger rating before eating ____ Hunger rating after eating ____

Dinner   ____:____   Hunger rating before eating ____ Hunger rating after eating ____

Did you meet your hunger scale goals?   Y   N

ACTIVITY LEVEL:　　0　1　2　3　4　5

Did you eat three meals and at least one snack, including a nutritious breakfast?　　Y　N

NOTES _____

_____

Eating cutoff time: ____:____　　　Bedtime: ____:____

Did you cut off eating at least two hours before bedtime?　　Y　N

NOTES _____

_____

Did you drink at least six 8-ounce glasses of water?　　Y　N

NOTES _____

_____

Did you abstain from alcohol?　　Y　N

NOTES _____

_____

Did you take your vitamin supplements?　　Y　N

NOTES _____

_____

Aerobic minutes or steps/day _____

Did you meet your goal?　　Y　N

NOTES _____

_____

STRENGTH TRAINING

Exercise								
Weight								
Reps								
Sets								

Breakfast ____:____　Hunger rating before eating ____ Hunger rating after eating ____

Lunch　　____:____　Hunger rating before eating ____ Hunger rating after eating ____

Dinner　　____:____　Hunger rating before eating ____ Hunger rating after eating ____

Did you meet your hunger scale goals?　　Y　N

ACTIVITY LEVEL: 0   1   2   3   4   5

Did you eat three meals and at least one snack, including a nutritious breakfast?   Y   N
NOTES _____

_____

Eating cutoff time: ____:____   Bedtime: ____:____
Did you cut off eating at least two hours before bedtime?   Y   N
NOTES _____

_____

Did you drink at least six 8-ounce glasses of water?   Y   N
NOTES _____

_____

Did you abstain from alcohol?   Y   N
NOTES _____

_____

Did you take your vitamin supplements?   Y   N
NOTES _____

_____

Aerobic minutes or steps/day _____
Did you meet your goal?   Y   N
NOTES _____

_____

STRENGTH TRAINING

Exercise								
Weight								
Reps								
Sets								

Breakfast   ____:____   Hunger rating before eating ____   Hunger rating after eating ____

Lunch   ____:____   Hunger rating before eating ____   Hunger rating after eating ____

Dinner   ____:____   Hunger rating before eating ____   Hunger rating after eating ____

Did you meet your hunger scale goals?   Y   N

ACTIVITY LEVEL: 0   1   2   3   4   5

Did you eat three meals and at least one snack, including a nutritious breakfast?   Y   N
NOTES_____
_____

Eating cutoff time: ____:____   Bedtime: ____:____

Did you cut off eating at least two hours before bedtime?   Y   N
NOTES_____
_____

Did you drink at least six 8-ounce glasses of water?   Y   N
NOTES_____
_____

Did you abstain from alcohol?   Y   N
NOTES_____
_____

Did you take your vitamin supplements?   Y   N
NOTES_____
_____

Aerobic minutes or steps/day _____
Did you meet your goal?   Y   N
NOTES_____
_____

STRENGTH TRAINING

Exercise								
Weight								
Reps								
Sets								

Breakfast   ____:____   Hunger rating before eating ____   Hunger rating after eating ____

Lunch   ____:____   Hunger rating before eating ____   Hunger rating after eating ____

Dinner   ____:____   Hunger rating before eating ____   Hunger rating after eating ____

Did you meet your hunger scale goals?   Y   N

WEEK: **DATE:**   **PHASE 2**

ACTIVITY LEVEL: 0   1   2   3   4   5

Did you eat three meals and at least one snack, including a nutritious breakfast?   Y   N
NOTES _____
_____

Eating cutoff time: ____:____   Bedtime: ____:____
Did you cut off eating at least two hours before bedtime?   Y   N
NOTES _____
_____

Did you drink at least six 8-ounce glasses of water?   Y   N
NOTES _____
_____

Did you abstain from alcohol?   Y   N
NOTES _____
_____

Did you take your vitamin supplements?   Y   N
NOTES _____
_____

Aerobic minutes or steps/day _____
Did you meet your goal?   Y   N
NOTES _____
_____

STRENGTH TRAINING

Exercise								
Weight								
Reps								
Sets								

Breakfast   ____:____   Hunger rating before eating ____ Hunger rating after eating ____
Lunch   ____:____   Hunger rating before eating ____ Hunger rating after eating ____
Dinner   ____:____   Hunger rating before eating ____ Hunger rating after eating ____
Did you meet your hunger scale goals?   Y   N

ACTIVITY LEVEL: 0   1   2   3   4   5

Did you eat three meals and at least one snack, including a nutritious breakfast?   Y   N

NOTES _____

_____

Eating cutoff time: ____:____   Bedtime: ____:____

Did you cut off eating at least two hours before bedtime?   Y   N

NOTES _____

_____

Did you drink at least six 8-ounce glasses of water?   Y   N

NOTES _____

_____

Did you abstain from alcohol?   Y   N

NOTES _____

_____

Did you take your vitamin supplements?   Y   N

NOTES _____

_____

Aerobic minutes or steps/day _____

Did you meet your goal?   Y   N

NOTES _____

_____

STRENGTH TRAINING

Exercise								
Weight								
Reps								
Sets								

Breakfast ____:____   Hunger rating before eating ____ Hunger rating after eating ____

Lunch   ____:____   Hunger rating before eating ____ Hunger rating after eating ____

Dinner   ____:____   Hunger rating before eating ____ Hunger rating after eating ____

Did you meet your hunger scale goals?   Y   N

ACTIVITY LEVEL: 0   1   2   3   4   5

Did you eat three meals and at least one snack, including a nutritious breakfast?   Y   N

NOTES _____

_____

Eating cutoff time: ____:____   Bedtime: ____:____

Did you cut off eating at least two hours before bedtime?   Y   N

NOTES _____

_____

Did you drink at least six 8-ounce glasses of water?   Y   N

NOTES _____

_____

Did you abstain from alcohol?   Y   N

NOTES _____

_____

Did you take your vitamin supplements?   Y   N

NOTES _____

_____

Aerobic minutes or steps/day _____

Did you meet your goal?   Y   N

NOTES _____

_____

STRENGTH TRAINING

Exercise								
Weight								
Reps								
Sets								

Breakfast   ____:____   Hunger rating before eating ____ Hunger rating after eating ____

Lunch   ____:____   Hunger rating before eating ____ Hunger rating after eating ____

Dinner   ____:____   Hunger rating before eating ____ Hunger rating after eating ____

Did you meet your hunger scale goals?   Y   N

Weekly Summary

Your weight: _____

How many days did you eat three meals and at least one snack? _____

How many days did you cut off your eating at least two hours before bedtime? _____

How many days did you drink at least six 8-ounce glasses of water? _____

How many days did you abstain from alcohol? _____

How many days did you take your vitamin supplements? _____

Total aerobic minutes/steps for the week _____

Did you meet your aerobic/step goal?   Y   N

Did you meet your strength training goals for the week?   Y   N

How was your week overall? _____

_____

_____

_____

_____

_____

_____

_____

_____

_____

_____

_____

_____

_____

_____

_____

_____

_____

_____

_____

_____

ACTIVITY LEVEL: 0   1   2   3   4   5

Did you eat three meals and at least one snack, including a nutritious breakfast?   Y   N
NOTES _____
_____

Eating cutoff time: ____:____   Bedtime: ____:____
Did you cut off eating at least two hours before bedtime?   Y   N
NOTES _____
_____

Did you drink at least six 8-ounce glasses of water?   Y   N
NOTES _____
_____

Did you abstain from alcohol?   Y   N
NOTES _____
_____

Did you take your vitamin supplements?   Y   N
NOTES _____
_____

Aerobic minutes or steps/day _____
Did you meet your goal?   Y   N
NOTES _____
_____

STRENGTH TRAINING

Exercise								
Weight								
Reps								
Sets								

Breakfast ____:____ Hunger rating before eating ____ Hunger rating after eating ____

Lunch ____:____ Hunger rating before eating ____ Hunger rating after eating ____

Dinner ____:____ Hunger rating before eating ____ Hunger rating after eating ____

Did you meet your hunger scale goals?   Y   N

ACTIVITY LEVEL: 0   1   2   3   4   5

Did you eat three meals and at least one snack, including a nutritious breakfast?   Y   N
NOTES _____
_____

Eating cutoff time: ____:____   Bedtime: ____:____
Did you cut off eating at least two hours before bedtime?   Y   N
NOTES _____
_____

Did you drink at least six 8-ounce glasses of water?   Y   N
NOTES _____
_____

Did you abstain from alcohol?   Y   N
NOTES _____
_____

Did you take your vitamin supplements?   Y   N
NOTES _____
_____

Aerobic minutes or steps/day _____
Did you meet your goal?   Y   N
NOTES _____
_____

STRENGTH TRAINING

Exercise								
Weight								
Reps								
Sets								

Breakfast   ____:____   Hunger rating before eating ____ Hunger rating after eating ____

Lunch   ____:____   Hunger rating before eating ____ Hunger rating after eating ____

Dinner   ____:____   Hunger rating before eating ____ Hunger rating after eating ____

Did you meet your hunger scale goals?   Y   N

ACTIVITY LEVEL: 0 1 2 3 4 5

Did you eat three meals and at least one snack, including a nutritious breakfast?   Y N

NOTES _____

_____

Eating cutoff time: ___:___   Bedtime: ___:___

Did you cut off eating at least two hours before bedtime?   Y N

NOTES _____

_____

Did you drink at least six 8-ounce glasses of water?   Y N

NOTES _____

_____

Did you abstain from alcohol?   Y N

NOTES _____

_____

Did you take your vitamin supplements?   Y N

NOTES _____

_____

Aerobic minutes or steps/day _____

Did you meet your goal?   Y N

NOTES _____

_____

STRENGTH TRAINING

Exercise								
Weight								
Reps								
Sets								

Breakfast ___:___   Hunger rating before eating ____ Hunger rating after eating ____

Lunch ___:___   Hunger rating before eating ____ Hunger rating after eating ____

Dinner ___:___   Hunger rating before eating ____ Hunger rating after eating ____

Did you meet your hunger scale goals?   Y N

ACTIVITY LEVEL: 0   1   2   3   4   5

Did you eat three meals and at least one snack, including a nutritious breakfast?   Y   N

NOTES _____

_____

Eating cutoff time: ____:____   Bedtime: ____:____

Did you cut off eating at least two hours before bedtime?   Y   N

NOTES _____

_____

Did you drink at least six 8-ounce glasses of water?   Y   N

NOTES _____

_____

Did you abstain from alcohol?   Y   N

NOTES _____

_____

Did you take your vitamin supplements?   Y   N

NOTES _____

_____

Aerobic minutes or steps/day _____

Did you meet your goal?   Y   N

NOTES _____

_____

STRENGTH TRAINING

Exercise								
Weight								
Reps								
Sets								

Breakfast ____:____   Hunger rating before eating ____   Hunger rating after eating ____

Lunch ____:____   Hunger rating before eating ____   Hunger rating after eating ____

Dinner ____:____   Hunger rating before eating ____   Hunger rating after eating ____

Did you meet your hunger scale goals?   Y   N

ACTIVITY LEVEL:　　0　1　2　3　4　5

Did you eat three meals and at least one snack, including a nutritious breakfast?　　Y　N

NOTES _____

_____

Eating cutoff time: ____:____　　　　Bedtime: ____:____

Did you cut off eating at least two hours before bedtime?　　Y　N

NOTES _____

_____

Did you drink at least six 8-ounce glasses of water?　　Y　N

NOTES _____

_____

Did you abstain from alcohol?　　Y　N

NOTES _____

_____

Did you take your vitamin supplements?　　Y　N

NOTES _____

_____

Aerobic minutes or steps/day _____

Did you meet your goal?　　Y　N

NOTES _____

_____

STRENGTH TRAINING

Exercise								
Weight								
Reps								
Sets								

Breakfast ____:____ Hunger rating before eating ____ Hunger rating after eating ____

Lunch ____:____ Hunger rating before eating ____ Hunger rating after eating ____

Dinner ____:____ Hunger rating before eating ____ Hunger rating after eating ____

Did you meet your hunger scale goals?　　Y　N

ACTIVITY LEVEL: 0   1   2   3   4   5

Did you eat three meals and at least one snack, including a nutritious breakfast?   Y   N
NOTES _____
_____

Eating cutoff time: ____:____   Bedtime: ____:____
Did you cut off eating at least two hours before bedtime?   Y   N
NOTES _____
_____

Did you drink at least six 8-ounce glasses of water?   Y   N
NOTES _____
_____

Did you abstain from alcohol?   Y   N
NOTES _____
_____

Did you take your vitamin supplements?   Y   N
NOTES _____
_____

Aerobic minutes or steps/day _____
Did you meet your goal?   Y   N
NOTES _____
_____

STRENGTH TRAINING

Exercise							
Weight							
Reps							
Sets							

Breakfast ____:____   Hunger rating before eating ____ Hunger rating after eating ____

Lunch   ____:____   Hunger rating before eating ____ Hunger rating after eating ____

Dinner   ____:____   Hunger rating before eating ____ Hunger rating after eating ____

Did you meet your hunger scale goals?   Y   N

ACTIVITY LEVEL:　0　1　2　3　4　5

Did you eat three meals and at least one snack, including a nutritious breakfast?　　Y　N
NOTES _____
_____

Eating cutoff time: ___:___　　　　Bedtime: ___:___
Did you cut off eating at least two hours before bedtime?　　Y　N
NOTES _____
_____

Did you drink at least six 8-ounce glasses of water?　　Y　N
NOTES _____
_____

Did you abstain from alcohol?　　Y　N
NOTES _____
_____

Did you take your vitamin supplements?　　Y　N
NOTES _____
_____

Aerobic minutes or steps/day _____
Did you meet your goal?　　Y　N
NOTES _____
_____

STRENGTH TRAINING

Exercise								
Weight								
Reps								
Sets								

Breakfast ___:___　Hunger rating before eating ____ Hunger rating after eating ____

Lunch ___:___　Hunger rating before eating ____ Hunger rating after eating ____

Dinner ___:___　Hunger rating before eating ____ Hunger rating after eating ____

Did you meet your hunger scale goals?　　Y　N

Weekly Summary

Your weight: _____

How many days did you eat three meals and at least one snack? _____

How many days did you cut off your eating at least two hours before bedtime? _____

How many days did you drink at least six 8-ounce glasses of water? _____

How many days did you abstain from alcohol? _____

How many days did you take your vitamin supplements? _____

Total aerobic minutes/steps for the week _____

Did you meet your aerobic/step goal?   Y   N

Did you meet your strength training goals for the week?   Y   N

How was your week overall? _____

_____

_____

_____

_____

_____

_____

_____

_____

_____

_____

_____

_____

_____

_____

_____

_____

_____

_____

_____

_____

_____

ACTIVITY LEVEL: 0   1   2   3   4   5

Did you eat three meals and at least one snack, including a nutritious breakfast?   Y   N
NOTES _____
_____

Eating cutoff time: ____:____   Bedtime: ____:____
Did you cut off eating at least two hours before bedtime?   Y   N
NOTES _____
_____

Did you drink at least six 8-ounce glasses of water?   Y   N
NOTES _____
_____

Did you abstain from alcohol?   Y   N
NOTES _____
_____

Did you take your vitamin supplements?   Y   N
NOTES _____
_____

Aerobic minutes or steps/day _____
Did you meet your goal?   Y   N
NOTES _____
_____

STRENGTH TRAINING

Exercise								
Weight								
Reps								
Sets								

Breakfast   ____:____   Hunger rating before eating ____ Hunger rating after eating ____

Lunch   ____:____   Hunger rating before eating ____ Hunger rating after eating ____

Dinner   ____:____   Hunger rating before eating ____ Hunger rating after eating ____

Did you meet your hunger scale goals?   Y   N

ACTIVITY LEVEL: 0   1   2   3   4   5

Did you eat three meals and at least one snack, including a nutritious breakfast?   Y   N
NOTES_____

_____

Eating cutoff time: ____:____   Bedtime: ____:____
Did you cut off eating at least two hours before bedtime?   Y   N
NOTES_____

_____

Did you drink at least six 8-ounce glasses of water?   Y   N
NOTES_____

_____

Did you abstain from alcohol?   Y   N
NOTES_____

_____

Did you take your vitamin supplements?   Y   N
NOTES_____

_____

Aerobic minutes or steps/day _____
Did you meet your goal?   Y   N
NOTES_____

_____

STRENGTH TRAINING

Exercise							
Weight							
Reps							
Sets							

Breakfast   ____:____   Hunger rating before eating ____ Hunger rating after eating ____

Lunch   ____:____   Hunger rating before eating ____ Hunger rating after eating ____

Dinner   ____:____   Hunger rating before eating ____ Hunger rating after eating ____

Did you meet your hunger scale goals?   Y   N

ACTIVITY LEVEL:　0　1　2　3　4　5

Did you eat three meals and at least one snack, including a nutritious breakfast?　　　Y　N
NOTES_____
_____

Eating cutoff time: ____:____　　　Bedtime: ____:____
Did you cut off eating at least two hours before bedtime?　　　Y　N
NOTES_____
_____

Did you drink at least six 8-ounce glasses of water?　　　Y　N
NOTES_____
_____

Did you abstain from alcohol?　　　Y　N
NOTES_____
_____

Did you take your vitamin supplements?　　　Y　N
NOTES_____
_____

Aerobic minutes or steps/day _____
Did you meet your goal?　　　Y　N
NOTES_____
_____

STRENGTH TRAINING

Exercise								
Weight								
Reps								
Sets								

Breakfast ____:____　Hunger rating before eating ____ Hunger rating after eating ____

Lunch ____:____　Hunger rating before eating ____ Hunger rating after eating ____

Dinner ____:____　Hunger rating before eating ____ Hunger rating after eating ____

Did you meet your hunger scale goals?　　　Y　N

ACTIVITY LEVEL: 0   1   2   3   4   5

Did you eat three meals and at least one snack, including a nutritious breakfast?   Y   N
NOTES_____
_____

Eating cutoff time: ____:____   Bedtime: ____:____
Did you cut off eating at least two hours before bedtime?   Y   N
NOTES_____
_____

Did you drink at least six 8-ounce glasses of water?   Y   N
NOTES_____
_____

Did you abstain from alcohol?   Y   N
NOTES_____
_____

Did you take your vitamin supplements?   Y   N
NOTES_____
_____

Aerobic minutes or steps/day _____
Did you meet your goal?   Y   N
NOTES_____
_____

STRENGTH TRAINING

Exercise								
Weight								
Reps								
Sets								

Breakfast   ____:____   Hunger rating before eating ____ Hunger rating after eating ____

Lunch   ____:____   Hunger rating before eating ____ Hunger rating after eating ____

Dinner   ____:____   Hunger rating before eating ____ Hunger rating after eating ____

Did you meet your hunger scale goals?   Y   N

ACTIVITY LEVEL: 0   1   2   3   4   5

Did you eat three meals and at least one snack, including a nutritious breakfast?   Y   N
NOTES_____

_____

Eating cutoff time: ____:____   Bedtime: ____:____
Did you cut off eating at least two hours before bedtime?   Y   N
NOTES_____

_____

Did you drink at least six 8-ounce glasses of water?   Y   N
NOTES_____

_____

Did you abstain from alcohol?   Y   N
NOTES_____

_____

Did you take your vitamin supplements?   Y   N
NOTES_____

_____

Aerobic minutes or steps/day _____
Did you meet your goal?   Y   N
NOTES_____

_____

STRENGTH TRAINING

Exercise								
Weight								
Reps								
Sets								

Breakfast ____:____   Hunger rating before eating ____ Hunger rating after eating ____

Lunch   ____:____   Hunger rating before eating ____ Hunger rating after eating ____

Dinner   ____:____   Hunger rating before eating ____ Hunger rating after eating ____

Did you meet your hunger scale goals?   Y   N

ACTIVITY LEVEL: 0 1 2 3 4 5

Did you eat three meals and at least one snack, including a nutritious breakfast? Y N
NOTES _____
_____

Eating cutoff time: ___:___ Bedtime: ___:___
Did you cut off eating at least two hours before bedtime? Y N
NOTES _____
_____

Did you drink at least six 8-ounce glasses of water? Y N
NOTES _____
_____

Did you abstain from alcohol? Y N
NOTES _____
_____

Did you take your vitamin supplements? Y N
NOTES _____
_____

Aerobic minutes or steps/day _____
Did you meet your goal? Y N
NOTES _____
_____

STRENGTH TRAINING

Exercise								
Weight								
Reps								
Sets								

Breakfast ___:___ Hunger rating before eating ____ Hunger rating after eating ____

Lunch ___:___ Hunger rating before eating ____ Hunger rating after eating ____

Dinner ___:___ Hunger rating before eating ____ Hunger rating after eating ____

Did you meet your hunger scale goals? Y N

ACTIVITY LEVEL: 0   1   2   3   4   5

Did you eat three meals and at least one snack, including a nutritious breakfast?   Y   N

NOTES _____

_____

Eating cutoff time: ____:____   Bedtime: ____:____

Did you cut off eating at least two hours before bedtime?   Y   N

NOTES _____

_____

Did you drink at least six 8-ounce glasses of water?   Y   N

NOTES _____

_____

Did you abstain from alcohol?   Y   N

NOTES _____

_____

Did you take your vitamin supplements?   Y   N

NOTES _____

_____

Aerobic minutes or steps/day _____

Did you meet your goal?   Y   N

NOTES _____

_____

STRENGTH TRAINING

Exercise								
Weight								
Reps								
Sets								

Breakfast   ____:____   Hunger rating before eating ____   Hunger rating after eating ____

Lunch   ____:____   Hunger rating before eating ____   Hunger rating after eating ____

Dinner   ____:____   Hunger rating before eating ____   Hunger rating after eating ____

Did you meet your hunger scale goals?   Y   N

Weekly Summary

Your weight: _____

How many days did you eat three meals and at least one snack?   _____

How many days did you cut off your eating at least two hours before bedtime?   _____

How many days did you drink at least six 8-ounce glasses of water?   _____

How many days did you abstain from alcohol?   _____

How many days did you take your vitamin supplements?   _____

Total aerobic minutes/steps for the week   _____

Did you meet your aerobic/step goal?   Y N

Did you meet your strength training goals for the week?   Y N

How was your week overall? _____

_____

_____

_____

_____

_____

_____

_____

_____

_____

_____

_____

_____

_____

_____

_____

_____

_____

_____

_____

_____

_____

ACTIVITY LEVEL: 0   1   2   3   4   5

Did you eat three meals and at least one snack, including a nutritious breakfast?   Y   N
NOTES _____
_____

Eating cutoff time: ___:___   Bedtime: ___:___
Did you cut off eating at least two hours before bedtime?   Y   N
NOTES _____
_____

Did you drink at least six 8-ounce glasses of water?   Y   N
NOTES _____
_____

Did you abstain from alcohol?   Y   N
NOTES _____
_____

Did you take your vitamin supplements?   Y   N
NOTES _____
_____

Aerobic minutes or steps/day _____
Did you meet your goal?   Y   N
NOTES _____
_____

STRENGTH TRAINING

Exercise								
Weight								
Reps								
Sets								

Breakfast ___:___   Hunger rating before eating ____ Hunger rating after eating ____

Lunch   ___:___   Hunger rating before eating ____ Hunger rating after eating ____

Dinner   ___:___   Hunger rating before eating ____ Hunger rating after eating ____

Did you meet your hunger scale goals?   Y   N

ACTIVITY LEVEL: 0   1   2   3   4   5

Did you eat three meals and at least one snack, including a nutritious breakfast?   Y   N
NOTES _____

_____

Eating cutoff time: ____:____   Bedtime: ____:____

Did you cut off eating at least two hours before bedtime?   Y   N
NOTES _____

_____

Did you drink at least six 8-ounce glasses of water?   Y   N
NOTES _____

_____

Did you abstain from alcohol?   Y   N
NOTES _____

_____

Did you take your vitamin supplements?   Y   N
NOTES _____

_____

Aerobic minutes or steps/day _____

Did you meet your goal?   Y   N
NOTES _____

_____

STRENGTH TRAINING

Exercise								
Weight								
Reps								
Sets								

Breakfast   ____:____   Hunger rating before eating ____ Hunger rating after eating ____

Lunch   ____:____   Hunger rating before eating ____ Hunger rating after eating ____

Dinner   ____:____   Hunger rating before eating ____ Hunger rating after eating ____

Did you meet your hunger scale goals?   Y   N

ACTIVITY LEVEL: 0   1   2   3   4   5

Did you eat three meals and at least one snack, including a nutritious breakfast?   Y   N
NOTES_____
_____

Eating cutoff time: ____:____   Bedtime: ____:____
Did you cut off eating at least two hours before bedtime?   Y   N
NOTES_____
_____

Did you drink at least six 8-ounce glasses of water?   Y   N
NOTES_____
_____

Did you abstain from alcohol?   Y   N
NOTES_____
_____

Did you take your vitamin supplements?   Y   N
NOTES_____
_____

Aerobic minutes or steps/day _____
Did you meet your goal?   Y   N
NOTES_____
_____

STRENGTH TRAINING

Exercise								
Weight								
Reps								
Sets								

Breakfast   ____:____   Hunger rating before eating ____ Hunger rating after eating ____
Lunch   ____:____   Hunger rating before eating ____ Hunger rating after eating ____
Dinner   ____:____   Hunger rating before eating ____ Hunger rating after eating ____

Did you meet your hunger scale goals?   Y   N

ACTIVITY LEVEL: 0   1   2   3   4   5

Did you eat three meals and at least one snack, including a nutritious breakfast?   Y   N
NOTES _____

_____

Eating cutoff time: ____:____   Bedtime: ____:____

Did you cut off eating at least two hours before bedtime?   Y   N
NOTES _____

_____

Did you drink at least six 8-ounce glasses of water?   Y   N
NOTES _____

_____

Did you abstain from alcohol?   Y   N
NOTES _____

_____

Did you take your vitamin supplements?   Y   N
NOTES _____

_____

Aerobic minutes or steps/day _____

Did you meet your goal?   Y   N
NOTES _____

_____

STRENGTH TRAINING

Exercise								
Weight								
Reps								
Sets								

Breakfast   ____:____   Hunger rating before eating ____   Hunger rating after eating ____

Lunch   ____:____   Hunger rating before eating ____   Hunger rating after eating ____

Dinner   ____:____   Hunger rating before eating ____   Hunger rating after eating ____

Did you meet your hunger scale goals?   Y   N

ACTIVITY LEVEL: 0   1   2   3   4   5

Did you eat three meals and at least one snack, including a nutritious breakfast?   Y   N
NOTES _____
_____

Eating cutoff time: ____:____   Bedtime: ____:____
Did you cut off eating at least two hours before bedtime?   Y   N
NOTES _____
_____

Did you drink at least six 8-ounce glasses of water?   Y   N
NOTES _____
_____

Did you abstain from alcohol?   Y   N
NOTES _____
_____

Did you take your vitamin supplements?   Y   N
NOTES _____
_____

Aerobic minutes or steps/day _____
Did you meet your goal?   Y   N
NOTES _____
_____

STRENGTH TRAINING

Exercise								
Weight								
Reps								
Sets								

Breakfast   ____:____   Hunger rating before eating ____ Hunger rating after eating ____

Lunch   ____:____   Hunger rating before eating ____ Hunger rating after eating ____

Dinner   ____:____   Hunger rating before eating ____ Hunger rating after eating ____

Did you meet your hunger scale goals?   Y   N

ACTIVITY LEVEL: 0   1   2   3   4   5

Did you eat three meals and at least one snack, including a nutritious breakfast?   Y   N

NOTES _____

_____

Eating cutoff time: ____:____   Bedtime: ____:____

Did you cut off eating at least two hours before bedtime?   Y   N

NOTES _____

_____

Did you drink at least six 8-ounce glasses of water?   Y   N

NOTES _____

_____

Did you abstain from alcohol?   Y   N

NOTES _____

_____

Did you take your vitamin supplements?   Y   N

NOTES _____

_____

Aerobic minutes or steps/day _____

Did you meet your goal?   Y   N

NOTES _____

_____

STRENGTH TRAINING

Exercise								
Weight								
Reps								
Sets								

Breakfast ____:____   Hunger rating before eating ____ Hunger rating after eating ____

Lunch   ____:____   Hunger rating before eating ____ Hunger rating after eating ____

Dinner   ____:____   Hunger rating before eating ____ Hunger rating after eating ____

Did you meet your hunger scale goals?   Y   N

ACTIVITY LEVEL: 0   1   2   3   4   5

Did you eat three meals and at least one snack, including a nutritious breakfast?   Y   N
NOTES _____
_____

Eating cutoff time: ____:____   Bedtime: ____:____
Did you cut off eating at least two hours before bedtime?   Y   N
NOTES _____
_____

Did you drink at least six 8-ounce glasses of water?   Y   N
NOTES _____
_____

Did you abstain from alcohol?   Y   N
NOTES _____
_____

Did you take your vitamin supplements?   Y   N
NOTES _____
_____

Aerobic minutes or steps/day _____
Did you meet your goal?   Y   N
NOTES _____
_____

STRENGTH TRAINING

Exercise								
Weight								
Reps								
Sets								

Breakfast ____:____   Hunger rating before eating ____   Hunger rating after eating ____

Lunch   ____:____   Hunger rating before eating ____   Hunger rating after eating ____

Dinner   ____:____   Hunger rating before eating ____   Hunger rating after eating ____

Did you meet your hunger scale goals?   Y   N

Weekly Summary

Your weight: _____

How many days did you eat three meals and at least one snack? _____

How many days did you cut off your eating at least two hours before bedtime? _____

How many days did you drink at least six 8-ounce glasses of water? _____

How many days did you abstain from alcohol? _____

How many days did you take your vitamin supplements? _____

Total aerobic minutes/steps for the week _____

Did you meet your aerobic/step goal?   Y   N

Did you meet your strength training goals for the week?   Y   N

How was your week overall? _____

_____

_____

_____

_____

_____

_____

_____

_____

_____

_____

_____

_____

_____

_____

_____

_____

_____

_____

_____

_____

_____

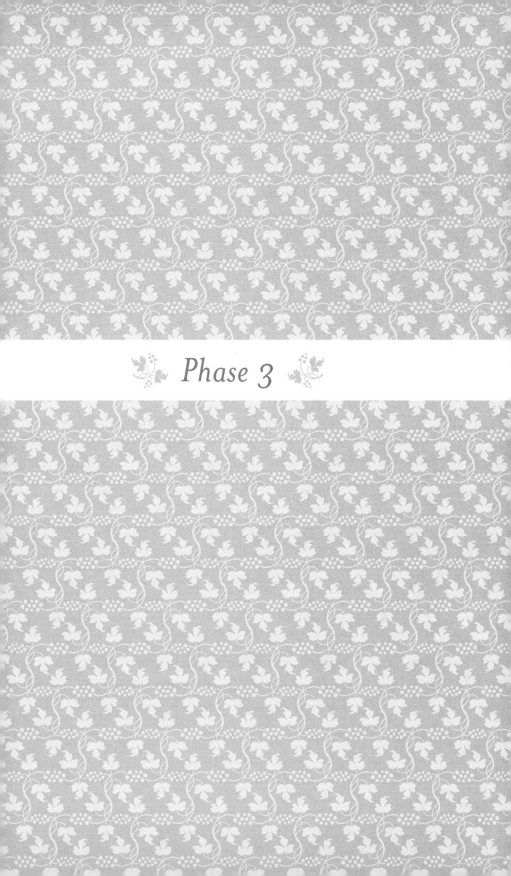

Phase 3

ACTIVITY LEVEL: 0   1   2   3   4   5

Did you eat three meals and at least one snack, including a nutritious breakfast?   Y   N

NOTES _____

_____

Eating cutoff time: ____:____   Bedtime: ____:____

Did you cut off eating at least two hours before bedtime?   Y   N

NOTES _____

_____

Did you drink at least six 8-ounce glasses of water?   Y   N

NOTES _____

_____

Did you abstain from alcohol?   Y   N

NOTES _____

_____

Did you take your vitamin supplements?   Y   N

NOTES _____

_____

Aerobic minutes or steps/day _____

Did you meet your goal?   Y   N

NOTES _____

_____

STRENGTH TRAINING

Exercise								
Weight								
Reps								
Sets								

Breakfast   ____:____   Hunger rating before eating ____ Hunger rating after eating ____

Lunch   ____:____   Hunger rating before eating ____ Hunger rating after eating ____

Dinner   ____:____   Hunger rating before eating ____ Hunger rating after eating ____

Did you meet your hunger scale goals?   Y   N

WEEK: DATE: **PHASE 3**

ACTIVITY LEVEL: 0   1   2   3   4   5

Did you eat three meals and at least one snack, including a nutritious breakfast?   Y   N
NOTES _____
_____

Eating cutoff time: ___:___   Bedtime: ___:___
Did you cut off eating at least two hours before bedtime?   Y   N
NOTES _____
_____

Did you drink at least six 8-ounce glasses of water?   Y   N
NOTES _____
_____

Did you abstain from alcohol?   Y   N
NOTES _____
_____

Did you take your vitamin supplements?   Y   N
NOTES _____
_____

Aerobic minutes or steps/day _____
Did you meet your goal?   Y   N
NOTES _____
_____

STRENGTH TRAINING

Exercise								
Weight								
Reps								
Sets								

Breakfast ___:___   Hunger rating before eating ____   Hunger rating after eating ____

Lunch ___:___   Hunger rating before eating ____   Hunger rating after eating ____

Dinner ___:___   Hunger rating before eating ____   Hunger rating after eating ____

Did you meet your hunger scale goals?   Y   N

ACTIVITY LEVEL: 0   1   2   3   4   5

Did you eat three meals and at least one snack, including a nutritious breakfast?   Y   N
NOTES _____
_____

Eating cutoff time: ____:____   Bedtime: ____:____
Did you cut off eating at least two hours before bedtime?   Y   N
NOTES _____
_____

Did you drink at least six 8-ounce glasses of water?   Y   N
NOTES _____
_____

Did you abstain from alcohol?   Y   N
NOTES _____
_____

Did you take your vitamin supplements?   Y   N
NOTES _____
_____

Aerobic minutes or steps/day _____
Did you meet your goal?   Y   N
NOTES _____
_____

STRENGTH TRAINING

Exercise								
Weight								
Reps								
Sets								

Breakfast   ____:____   Hunger rating before eating ____   Hunger rating after eating ____

Lunch   ____:____   Hunger rating before eating ____   Hunger rating after eating ____

Dinner   ____:____   Hunger rating before eating ____   Hunger rating after eating ____

Did you meet your hunger scale goals?   Y   N

ACTIVITY LEVEL: 0 1 2 3 4 5

Did you eat three meals and at least one snack, including a nutritious breakfast? Y N
NOTES _____

_____

Eating cutoff time: ___:___ Bedtime: ___:___

Did you cut off eating at least two hours before bedtime? Y N
NOTES _____

_____

Did you drink at least six 8-ounce glasses of water? Y N
NOTES _____

_____

Did you abstain from alcohol? Y N
NOTES _____

_____

Did you take your vitamin supplements? Y N
NOTES _____

_____

Aerobic minutes or steps/day _____

Did you meet your goal? Y N
NOTES _____

_____

STRENGTH TRAINING

Exercise								
Weight								
Reps								
Sets								

Breakfast ___:___ Hunger rating before eating ____ Hunger rating after eating ____

Lunch ___:___ Hunger rating before eating ____ Hunger rating after eating ____

Dinner ___:___ Hunger rating before eating ____ Hunger rating after eating ____

Did you meet your hunger scale goals? Y N

ACTIVITY LEVEL: 0   1   2   3   4   5

Did you eat three meals and at least one snack, including a nutritious breakfast?   Y   N

NOTES_____

_____

Eating cutoff time: ____:____   Bedtime: ____:____

Did you cut off eating at least two hours before bedtime?   Y   N

NOTES_____

_____

Did you drink at least six 8-ounce glasses of water?   Y   N

NOTES_____

_____

Did you abstain from alcohol?   Y   N

NOTES_____

_____

Did you take your vitamin supplements?   Y   N

NOTES_____

_____

Aerobic minutes or steps/day _____

Did you meet your goal?   Y   N

NOTES_____

_____

STRENGTH TRAINING

Exercise								
Weight								
Reps								
Sets								

Breakfast   ____:____   Hunger rating before eating ____ Hunger rating after eating ____

Lunch   ____:____   Hunger rating before eating ____ Hunger rating after eating ____

Dinner   ____:____   Hunger rating before eating ____ Hunger rating after eating ____

Did you meet your hunger scale goals?   Y   N

ACTIVITY LEVEL: 0   1   2   3   4   5

Did you eat three meals and at least one snack, including a nutritious breakfast?   Y   N
NOTES _____
_____

Eating cutoff time: ___:___   Bedtime: ___:___
Did you cut off eating at least two hours before bedtime?   Y   N
NOTES _____
_____

Did you drink at least six 8-ounce glasses of water?   Y   N
NOTES _____
_____

Did you abstain from alcohol?   Y   N
NOTES _____
_____

Did you take your vitamin supplements?   Y   N
NOTES _____
_____

Aerobic minutes or steps/day _____
Did you meet your goal?   Y   N
NOTES _____
_____

STRENGTH TRAINING

Exercise								
Weight								
Reps								
Sets								

Breakfast   ___:___   Hunger rating before eating ____   Hunger rating after eating ____

Lunch   ___:___   Hunger rating before eating ____   Hunger rating after eating ____

Dinner   ___:___   Hunger rating before eating ____   Hunger rating after eating ____

Did you meet your hunger scale goals?   Y   N

ACTIVITY LEVEL: 0   1   2   3   4   5

Did you eat three meals and at least one snack, including a nutritious breakfast?   Y   N
NOTES_____

_____

Eating cutoff time: ____:____   Bedtime: ____:____

Did you cut off eating at least two hours before bedtime?   Y   N
NOTES_____

_____

Did you drink at least six 8-ounce glasses of water?   Y   N
NOTES_____

_____

Did you abstain from alcohol?   Y   N
NOTES_____

_____

Did you take your vitamin supplements?   Y   N
NOTES_____

_____

Aerobic minutes or steps/day _____

Did you meet your goal?   Y   N
NOTES_____

_____

STRENGTH TRAINING

Exercise								
Weight								
Reps								
Sets								

Breakfast ____:____   Hunger rating before eating ____ Hunger rating after eating ____

Lunch ____:____   Hunger rating before eating ____ Hunger rating after eating ____

Dinner ____:____   Hunger rating before eating ____ Hunger rating after eating ____

Did you meet your hunger scale goals?   Y   N

Weekly Summary

Your weight: _____

How many days did you eat three meals and at least one snack? _____

How many days did you cut off your eating at least two hours before bedtime? _____

How many days did you drink at least six 8-ounce glasses of water? _____

How many days did you abstain from alcohol? _____

How many days did you take your vitamin supplements? _____

Total aerobic minutes/steps for the week _____

Did you meet your aerobic/step goal?   Y   N

Did you meet your strength training goals for the week?   Y   N

How was your week overall? _____

_____

_____

_____

_____

_____

_____

_____

_____

_____

_____

_____

_____

_____

_____

_____

_____

_____

_____

_____

_____

_____

ACTIVITY LEVEL: 0   1   2   3   4   5

Did you eat three meals and at least one snack, including a nutritious breakfast?   Y   N
NOTES _____

_____

Eating cutoff time: ___:___   Bedtime: ___:___

Did you cut off eating at least two hours before bedtime?   Y   N
NOTES _____

_____

Did you drink at least six 8-ounce glasses of water?   Y   N
NOTES _____

_____

Did you abstain from alcohol?   Y   N
NOTES _____

_____

Did you take your vitamin supplements?   Y   N
NOTES _____

_____

Aerobic minutes or steps/day _____

Did you meet your goal?   Y   N
NOTES _____

_____

STRENGTH TRAINING

Exercise							
Weight							
Reps							
Sets							

Breakfast   ___:___   Hunger rating before eating ____ Hunger rating after eating ____

Lunch   ___:___   Hunger rating before eating ____ Hunger rating after eating ____

Dinner   ___:___   Hunger rating before eating ____ Hunger rating after eating ____

Did you meet your hunger scale goals?   Y   N

ACTIVITY LEVEL: 0   1   2   3   4   5

Did you eat three meals and at least one snack, including a nutritious breakfast?   Y   N
NOTES_____
_____

Eating cutoff time: ____:____   Bedtime: ____:____
Did you cut off eating at least two hours before bedtime?   Y   N
NOTES_____
_____

Did you drink at least six 8-ounce glasses of water?   Y   N
NOTES_____
_____

Did you abstain from alcohol?   Y   N
NOTES_____
_____

Did you take your vitamin supplements?   Y   N
NOTES_____
_____

Aerobic minutes or steps/day _____
Did you meet your goal?   Y   N
NOTES_____
_____

STRENGTH TRAINING

Exercise								
Weight								
Reps								
Sets								

Breakfast   ____:____   Hunger rating before eating ____   Hunger rating after eating ____

Lunch   ____:____   Hunger rating before eating ____   Hunger rating after eating ____

Dinner   ____:____   Hunger rating before eating ____   Hunger rating after eating ____

Did you meet your hunger scale goals?   Y   N

ACTIVITY LEVEL: 0   1   2   3   4   5

Did you eat three meals and at least one snack, including a nutritious breakfast?   Y   N
NOTES _____
_____

Eating cutoff time: ____:____   Bedtime: ____:____

Did you cut off eating at least two hours before bedtime?   Y   N
NOTES _____
_____

Did you drink at least six 8-ounce glasses of water?   Y   N
NOTES _____
_____

Did you abstain from alcohol?   Y   N
NOTES _____
_____

Did you take your vitamin supplements?   Y   N
NOTES _____
_____

Aerobic minutes or steps/day _____

Did you meet your goal?   Y   N
NOTES _____
_____

STRENGTH TRAINING

Exercise								
Weight								
Reps								
Sets								

Breakfast ____:____   Hunger rating before eating ____ Hunger rating after eating ____

Lunch   ____:____   Hunger rating before eating ____ Hunger rating after eating ____

Dinner   ____:____   Hunger rating before eating ____ Hunger rating after eating ____

Did you meet your hunger scale goals?   Y   N

WEEK: **DATE:**   **PHASE 3**

ACTIVITY LEVEL: 0   1   2   3   4   5

Did you eat three meals and at least one snack, including a nutritious breakfast?   Y   N
NOTES _____
_____

Eating cutoff time: ___:___   Bedtime: ___:___
Did you cut off eating at least two hours before bedtime?   Y   N
NOTES _____
_____

Did you drink at least six 8-ounce glasses of water?   Y   N
NOTES _____
_____

Did you abstain from alcohol?   Y   N
NOTES _____
_____

Did you take your vitamin supplements?   Y   N
NOTES _____
_____

Aerobic minutes or steps/day _____
Did you meet your goal?   Y   N
NOTES _____
_____

STRENGTH TRAINING

Exercise								
Weight								
Reps								
Sets								

Breakfast ___:___   Hunger rating before eating ____ Hunger rating after eating ____

Lunch   ___:___   Hunger rating before eating ____ Hunger rating after eating ____

Dinner   ___:___   Hunger rating before eating ____ Hunger rating after eating ____

Did you meet your hunger scale goals?   Y   N

WEEK: **DATE:**   **PHASE 3**

ACTIVITY LEVEL: 0   1   2   3   4   5

Did you eat three meals and at least one snack, including a nutritious breakfast?   Y   N
NOTES _____
_____

Eating cutoff time: ____:____   Bedtime: ____:____
Did you cut off eating at least two hours before bedtime?   Y   N
NOTES _____
_____

Did you drink at least six 8-ounce glasses of water?   Y   N
NOTES _____
_____

Did you abstain from alcohol?   Y   N
NOTES _____
_____

Did you take your vitamin supplements?   Y   N
NOTES _____
_____

Aerobic minutes or steps/day _____
Did you meet your goal?   Y   N
NOTES _____
_____

STRENGTH TRAINING

Exercise								
Weight								
Reps								
Sets								

Breakfast   ____:____   Hunger rating before eating ____   Hunger rating after eating ____

Lunch   ____:____   Hunger rating before eating ____   Hunger rating after eating ____

Dinner   ____:____   Hunger rating before eating ____   Hunger rating after eating ____

Did you meet your hunger scale goals?   Y   N

ACTIVITY LEVEL: 0   1   2   3   4   5

Did you eat three meals and at least one snack, including a nutritious breakfast?   Y   N
NOTES _____
_____

Eating cutoff time: ___:___   Bedtime: ___:___
Did you cut off eating at least two hours before bedtime?   Y   N
NOTES _____
_____

Did you drink at least six 8-ounce glasses of water?   Y   N
NOTES _____
_____

Did you abstain from alcohol?   Y   N
NOTES _____
_____

Did you take your vitamin supplements?   Y   N
NOTES _____
_____

Aerobic minutes or steps/day _____
Did you meet your goal?   Y   N
NOTES _____
_____

STRENGTH TRAINING

Exercise								
Weight								
Reps								
Sets								

Breakfast   ___:___   Hunger rating before eating ____ Hunger rating after eating ____
Lunch   ___:___   Hunger rating before eating ____ Hunger rating after eating ____
Dinner   ___:___   Hunger rating before eating ____ Hunger rating after eating ____

Did you meet your hunger scale goals?   Y   N

ACTIVITY LEVEL: 0   1   2   3   4   5

Did you eat three meals and at least one snack, including a nutritious breakfast?   Y   N
NOTES _____
_____

Eating cutoff time: ____:____   Bedtime: ____:____
Did you cut off eating at least two hours before bedtime?   Y   N
NOTES _____
_____

Did you drink at least six 8-ounce glasses of water?   Y   N
NOTES _____
_____

Did you abstain from alcohol?   Y   N
NOTES _____
_____

Did you take your vitamin supplements?   Y   N
NOTES _____
_____

Aerobic minutes or steps/day _____
Did you meet your goal?   Y   N
NOTES _____
_____

STRENGTH TRAINING

Exercise								
Weight								
Reps								
Sets								

Breakfast   ____:____   Hunger rating before eating ____ Hunger rating after eating ____

Lunch   ____:____   Hunger rating before eating ____ Hunger rating after eating ____

Dinner   ____:____   Hunger rating before eating ____ Hunger rating after eating ____

Did you meet your hunger scale goals?   Y   N

Weekly Summary

Your weight: _____

How many days did you eat three meals and at least one snack?   _____

How many days did you cut off your eating at least two hours before bedtime?   _____

How many days did you drink at least six 8-ounce glasses of water?   _____

How many days did you abstain from alcohol?   _____

How many days did you take your vitamin supplements?   _____

Total aerobic minutes/steps for the week   _____

Did you meet your aerobic/step goal?   Y   N

Did you meet your strength training goals for the week?   Y   N

How was your week overall? _____

_____

_____

_____

_____

_____

_____

_____

_____

_____

_____

_____

_____

_____

_____

_____

_____

_____

_____

_____

ACTIVITY LEVEL: 0   1   2   3   4   5

Did you eat three meals and at least one snack, including a nutritious breakfast?   Y   N
NOTES _____
_____

Eating cutoff time: ____:____   Bedtime: ____:____

Did you cut off eating at least two hours before bedtime?   Y   N
NOTES _____
_____

Did you drink at least six 8-ounce glasses of water?   Y   N
NOTES _____
_____

Did you abstain from alcohol?   Y   N
NOTES _____
_____

Did you take your vitamin supplements?   Y   N
NOTES _____
_____

Aerobic minutes or steps/day _____

Did you meet your goal?   Y   N
NOTES _____
_____

STRENGTH TRAINING

Exercise								
Weight								
Reps								
Sets								

Breakfast   ____:____   Hunger rating before eating ____   Hunger rating after eating ____

Lunch   ____:____   Hunger rating before eating ____   Hunger rating after eating ____

Dinner   ____:____   Hunger rating before eating ____   Hunger rating after eating ____

Did you meet your hunger scale goals?   Y   N

ACTIVITY LEVEL: 0   1   2   3   4   5

Did you eat three meals and at least one snack, including a nutritious breakfast?   Y   N
NOTES_____
_____

Eating cutoff time: ___:___   Bedtime: ___:___

Did you cut off eating at least two hours before bedtime?   Y   N
NOTES_____
_____

Did you drink at least six 8-ounce glasses of water?   Y   N
NOTES_____
_____

Did you abstain from alcohol?   Y   N
NOTES_____
_____

Did you take your vitamin supplements?   Y   N
NOTES_____
_____

Aerobic minutes or steps/day _____

Did you meet your goal?   Y   N
NOTES_____
_____

STRENGTH TRAINING

Exercise								
Weight								
Reps								
Sets								

Breakfast   ___:___   Hunger rating before eating ____ Hunger rating after eating ____

Lunch   ___:___   Hunger rating before eating ____ Hunger rating after eating ____

Dinner   ___:___   Hunger rating before eating ____ Hunger rating after eating ____

Did you meet your hunger scale goals?   Y   N

ACTIVITY LEVEL: 0   1   2   3   4   5

Did you eat three meals and at least one snack, including a nutritious breakfast?   Y   N
NOTES _____

_____

Eating cutoff time: ___:___   Bedtime: ___:___

Did you cut off eating at least two hours before bedtime?   Y   N
NOTES _____

_____

Did you drink at least six 8-ounce glasses of water?   Y   N
NOTES _____

_____

Did you abstain from alcohol?   Y   N
NOTES _____

_____

Did you take your vitamin supplements?   Y   N
NOTES _____

_____

Aerobic minutes or steps/day _____

Did you meet your goal?   Y   N
NOTES _____

_____

STRENGTH TRAINING

Exercise								
Weight								
Reps								
Sets								

Breakfast ___:___   Hunger rating before eating ____ Hunger rating after eating ____

Lunch   ___:___   Hunger rating before eating ____ Hunger rating after eating ____

Dinner   ___:___   Hunger rating before eating ____ Hunger rating after eating ____

Did you meet your hunger scale goals?   Y   N

ACTIVITY LEVEL: 0   1   2   3   4   5

Did you eat three meals and at least one snack, including a nutritious breakfast?   Y   N
NOTES _____
_____

Eating cutoff time: ____:____   Bedtime: ____:____
Did you cut off eating at least two hours before bedtime?   Y   N
NOTES _____
_____

Did you drink at least six 8-ounce glasses of water?   Y   N
NOTES _____
_____

Did you abstain from alcohol?   Y   N
NOTES _____
_____

Did you take your vitamin supplements?   Y   N
NOTES _____
_____

Aerobic minutes or steps/day _____
Did you meet your goal?   Y   N
NOTES _____
_____

STRENGTH TRAINING

Exercise								
Weight								
Reps								
Sets								

Breakfast   ____:____   Hunger rating before eating ____ Hunger rating after eating ____

Lunch   ____:____   Hunger rating before eating ____ Hunger rating after eating ____

Dinner   ____:____   Hunger rating before eating ____ Hunger rating after eating ____

Did you meet your hunger scale goals?   Y   N

ACTIVITY LEVEL: 0   1   2   3   4   5

Did you eat three meals and at least one snack, including a nutritious breakfast?   Y   N
NOTES _____

_____

Eating cutoff time: ____:____   Bedtime: ____:____

Did you cut off eating at least two hours before bedtime?   Y   N
NOTES _____

_____

Did you drink at least six 8-ounce glasses of water?   Y   N
NOTES _____

_____

Did you abstain from alcohol?   Y   N
NOTES _____

_____

Did you take your vitamin supplements?   Y   N
NOTES _____

_____

Aerobic minutes or steps/day _____

Did you meet your goal?   Y   N
NOTES _____

_____

STRENGTH TRAINING

Exercise								
Weight								
Reps								
Sets								

Breakfast   ____:____   Hunger rating before eating ____ Hunger rating after eating ____

Lunch   ____:____   Hunger rating before eating ____ Hunger rating after eating ____

Dinner   ____:____   Hunger rating before eating ____ Hunger rating after eating ____

Did you meet your hunger scale goals?   Y   N

ACTIVITY LEVEL: 0   1   2   3   4   5

Did you eat three meals and at least one snack, including a nutritious breakfast?   Y   N
NOTES_____
_____

Eating cutoff time: ___:___   Bedtime: ___:___
Did you cut off eating at least two hours before bedtime?   Y   N
NOTES_____
_____

Did you drink at least six 8-ounce glasses of water?   Y   N
NOTES_____
_____

Did you abstain from alcohol?   Y   N
NOTES_____
_____

Did you take your vitamin supplements?   Y   N
NOTES_____
_____

Aerobic minutes or steps/day _____
Did you meet your goal?   Y   N
NOTES_____
_____

STRENGTH TRAINING

Exercise								
Weight								
Reps								
Sets								

Breakfast ___:___ Hunger rating before eating ____ Hunger rating after eating ____
Lunch   ___:___ Hunger rating before eating ____ Hunger rating after eating ____
Dinner   ___:___ Hunger rating before eating ____ Hunger rating after eating ____

Did you meet your hunger scale goals?   Y   N

ACTIVITY LEVEL: 0   1   2   3   4   5

Did you eat three meals and at least one snack, including a nutritious breakfast?   Y   N
NOTES _____
_____

Eating cutoff time: ___:___   Bedtime: ___:___

Did you cut off eating at least two hours before bedtime?   Y   N
NOTES _____
_____

Did you drink at least six 8-ounce glasses of water?   Y   N
NOTES _____
_____

Did you abstain from alcohol?   Y   N
NOTES _____
_____

Did you take your vitamin supplements?   Y   N
NOTES _____
_____

Aerobic minutes or steps/day _____

Did you meet your goal?   Y   N
NOTES _____
_____

STRENGTH TRAINING

Exercise								
Weight								
Reps								
Sets								

Breakfast   ___:___   Hunger rating before eating ____ Hunger rating after eating ____

Lunch   ___:___   Hunger rating before eating ____ Hunger rating after eating ____

Dinner   ___:___   Hunger rating before eating ____ Hunger rating after eating ____

Did you meet your hunger scale goals?   Y   N

Weekly Summary

Your weight: _____

How many days did you eat three meals and at least one snack? _____

How many days did you cut off your eating at least two hours before bedtime? _____

How many days did you drink at least six 8-ounce glasses of water? _____

How many days did you abstain from alcohol? _____

How many days did you take your vitamin supplements? _____

Total aerobic minutes/steps for the week _____

Did you meet your aerobic/step goal?   Y   N

Did you meet your strength training goals for the week?   Y   N

How was your week overall? _____

_____

_____

_____

_____

_____

_____

_____

_____

_____

_____

_____

_____

_____

_____

_____

_____

_____

_____

_____

_____

_____

_____

_____

ACTIVITY LEVEL: 0   1   2   3   4   5

Did you eat three meals and at least one snack, including a nutritious breakfast?   Y   N
NOTES_____
_____

Eating cutoff time: ____:____   Bedtime: ____:____
Did you cut off eating at least two hours before bedtime?   Y   N
NOTES_____
_____

Did you drink at least six 8-ounce glasses of water?   Y   N
NOTES_____
_____

Did you abstain from alcohol?   Y   N
NOTES_____
_____

Did you take your vitamin supplements?   Y   N
NOTES_____
_____

Aerobic minutes or steps/day _____
Did you meet your goal?   Y   N
NOTES_____
_____

STRENGTH TRAINING

Exercise								
Weight								
Reps								
Sets								

Breakfast   ____:____   Hunger rating before eating ____ Hunger rating after eating ____

Lunch   ____:____   Hunger rating before eating ____ Hunger rating after eating ____

Dinner   ____:____   Hunger rating before eating ____ Hunger rating after eating ____

Did you meet your hunger scale goals?   Y   N

ACTIVITY LEVEL: 0   1   2   3   4   5

Did you eat three meals and at least one snack, including a nutritious breakfast?   Y   N
NOTES _____
_____

Eating cutoff time: ____:____   Bedtime: ____:____
Did you cut off eating at least two hours before bedtime?   Y   N
NOTES _____
_____

Did you drink at least six 8-ounce glasses of water?   Y   N
NOTES _____
_____

Did you abstain from alcohol?   Y   N
NOTES _____
_____

Did you take your vitamin supplements?   Y   N
NOTES _____
_____

Aerobic minutes or steps/day _____
Did you meet your goal?   Y   N
NOTES _____
_____

STRENGTH TRAINING

Exercise								
Weight								
Reps								
Sets								

Breakfast   ____:____   Hunger rating before eating ____ Hunger rating after eating ____

Lunch   ____:____   Hunger rating before eating ____ Hunger rating after eating ____

Dinner   ____:____   Hunger rating before eating ____ Hunger rating after eating ____

Did you meet your hunger scale goals?   Y   N

ACTIVITY LEVEL: 0   1   2   3   4   5

Did you eat three meals and at least one snack, including a nutritious breakfast?   Y   N

NOTES _____

_____

Eating cutoff time: ____:____   Bedtime: ____:____

Did you cut off eating at least two hours before bedtime?   Y   N

NOTES _____

_____

Did you drink at least six 8-ounce glasses of water?   Y   N

NOTES _____

_____

Did you abstain from alcohol?   Y   N

NOTES _____

_____

Did you take your vitamin supplements?   Y   N

NOTES _____

_____

Aerobic minutes or steps/day _____

Did you meet your goal?   Y   N

NOTES _____

_____

STRENGTH TRAINING

Exercise								
Weight								
Reps								
Sets								

Breakfast   ____:____   Hunger rating before eating ____   Hunger rating after eating ____

Lunch   ____:____   Hunger rating before eating ____   Hunger rating after eating ____

Dinner   ____:____   Hunger rating before eating ____   Hunger rating after eating ____

Did you meet your hunger scale goals?   Y   N

ACTIVITY LEVEL:　　0　1　2　3　4　5

Did you eat three meals and at least one snack, including a nutritious breakfast?　　Y　N
NOTES _____
_____

Eating cutoff time: ____:____　　　　Bedtime: ____:____
Did you cut off eating at least two hours before bedtime?　　Y　N
NOTES _____
_____

Did you drink at least six 8-ounce glasses of water?　　Y　N
NOTES _____
_____

Did you abstain from alcohol?　　Y　N
NOTES _____
_____

Did you take your vitamin supplements?　　Y　N
NOTES _____
_____

Aerobic minutes or steps/day _____
Did you meet your goal?　　Y　N
NOTES _____
_____

STRENGTH TRAINING

Exercise								
Weight								
Reps								
Sets								

Breakfast ____:____　Hunger rating before eating ____ Hunger rating after eating ____

Lunch ____:____　Hunger rating before eating ____ Hunger rating after eating ____

Dinner ____:____　Hunger rating before eating ____ Hunger rating after eating ____

Did you meet your hunger scale goals?　　Y　N

ACTIVITY LEVEL: 0   1   2   3   4   5

Did you eat three meals and at least one snack, including a nutritious breakfast?   Y   N
NOTES _____
_____

Eating cutoff time: ____:____   Bedtime: ____:____
Did you cut off eating at least two hours before bedtime?   Y   N
NOTES _____
_____

Did you drink at least six 8-ounce glasses of water?   Y   N
NOTES _____
_____

Did you abstain from alcohol?   Y   N
NOTES _____
_____

Did you take your vitamin supplements?   Y   N
NOTES _____
_____

Aerobic minutes or steps/day _____
Did you meet your goal?   Y   N
NOTES _____
_____

STRENGTH TRAINING

Exercise								
Weight								
Reps								
Sets								

Breakfast   ____:____   Hunger rating before eating ____ Hunger rating after eating ____

Lunch   ____:____   Hunger rating before eating ____ Hunger rating after eating ____

Dinner   ____:____   Hunger rating before eating ____ Hunger rating after eating ____

Did you meet your hunger scale goals?   Y   N

ACTIVITY LEVEL: 0   1   2   3   4   5

Did you eat three meals and at least one snack, including a nutritious breakfast?   Y   N

NOTES _____

_____

Eating cutoff time: ___:___   Bedtime: ___:___

Did you cut off eating at least two hours before bedtime?   Y   N

NOTES _____

_____

Did you drink at least six 8-ounce glasses of water?   Y   N

NOTES _____

_____

Did you abstain from alcohol?   Y   N

NOTES _____

_____

Did you take your vitamin supplements?   Y   N

NOTES _____

_____

Aerobic minutes or steps/day _____

Did you meet your goal?   Y   N

NOTES _____

_____

STRENGTH TRAINING

Exercise								
Weight								
Reps								
Sets								

Breakfast ___:___   Hunger rating before eating ____   Hunger rating after eating ____

Lunch   ___:___   Hunger rating before eating ____   Hunger rating after eating ____

Dinner   ___:___   Hunger rating before eating ____   Hunger rating after eating ____

Did you meet your hunger scale goals?   Y   N

ACTIVITY LEVEL: 0 1 2 3 4 5

Did you eat three meals and at least one snack, including a nutritious breakfast?　Y　N

NOTES_____

_____

Eating cutoff time: ___:___　　　Bedtime: ___:___

Did you cut off eating at least two hours before bedtime?　Y　N

NOTES_____

_____

Did you drink at least six 8-ounce glasses of water?　Y　N

NOTES_____

_____

Did you abstain from alcohol?　Y　N

NOTES_____

_____

Did you take your vitamin supplements?　Y　N

NOTES_____

_____

Aerobic minutes or steps/day _____

Did you meet your goal?　Y　N

NOTES_____

_____

STRENGTH TRAINING

Exercise								
Weight								
Reps								
Sets								

Breakfast ___:___　Hunger rating before eating ____　Hunger rating after eating ____

Lunch ___:___　Hunger rating before eating ____　Hunger rating after eating ____

Dinner ___:___　Hunger rating before eating ____　Hunger rating after eating ____

Did you meet your hunger scale goals?　Y　N

Weekly Summary

Your weight: _____

How many days did you eat three meals and at least one snack? _____

How many days did you cut off your eating at least two hours before bedtime? _____

How many days did you drink at least six 8-ounce glasses of water? _____

How many days did you abstain from alcohol? _____

How many days did you take your vitamin supplements? _____

Total aerobic minutes/steps for the week _____

Did you meet your aerobic/step goal?   Y   N

Did you meet your strength training goals for the week?   Y   N

How was your week overall? _____

_____

_____

_____

_____

_____

_____

_____

_____

_____

_____

_____

_____

_____

_____

_____

_____

_____

_____

_____

_____

_____

_____

Notes

Introducing Bob Greene's

bestlife™
thebestlife.com

Sign up today
for a 10-day Risk-FREE Trial
of the online diet plan

www.thebestlife.com/bookoffer

You'll Get:

1. Customized daily/weekly meal plans based on your lifestyle and preferences
2. Extensive Best Life approved recipe database
3. Online interaction with Bob Greene and his team of experts
4. Weekly feedback from Bob on your progress!
5. An interactive tool kit to help you put this book into action!